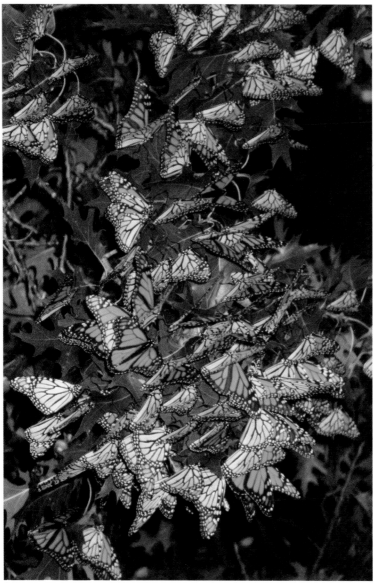

Minnesota Monarchs Courtesy of LoAnne Schluender

My
Personal Prayer
Journal

My
Personal Prayer
Journal

Doris Lyon

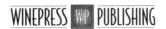
WINEPRESS WP PUBLISHING

ISBN 1-57921-173-9

9 781579 211738

Printed in the United States of America

Packaged by WinePress Publishing, PO Box 428, Enumclaw, WA 98022. The views expressed or implied in this work do not necessarily reflect those of WinePress Publishing. Ultimate design, content, and editorial accuracy of this work are the responsibilities of the author.

Unless otherwise noted all scriptures are taken from the Holy Bible, King James Version.

ISBN 1-57921-173-9

Contents

Get Acquainted with God through Prayer

Prayer is a private conversation between each of us and our heavenly Father; His Son Jesus, our Savior; and the Holy Spirit, our Comforter. The way directly to the throne of God is described in 1 Timothy 2:5: "For there is one God, and one mediator between God and men, the man Christ Jesus."

We are His special children, and we must use the special gifts He gives us—mainly receiving them through prayer. He wants us to have things, and He directs us how and what to pray for in many different verses in the Bible.

One direction is in Matthew 6:5–13. Verse 7 reads, "When ye pray, use not vain repetitions, as the heathen do: for they think that they will be heard for their much speaking." Matthew is saying, use your *own* words, telling God how things are with you. Your *own* words are precious to the Lord.

Do you know how you feel when you get a form letter in reply to your correspondence? God has those same feelings toward people rattling off memorized prayers without thinking about what they are saying. You don't memorize your side of the conversation with anyone else. Why do it with God?

In our country today, we need an intense revival of personal prayer in the proper direction. This manual is offered to help you have a more powerful prayer life. It will also help in counting your blessings and answers to prayers, thanking God, and giving Him glory and praise. Let us rejoice and praise Him for giving us this glorious opportunity! Let us use it constantly, as He has commanded us. 1 Thessalonians 5:17 says, "Pray without ceasing." We must learn how to do that.

This book is designed to

- Help us thank God for all our blessings, great and small
- Help us pray in a pleasing manner
- Help us remember what we prayed for
- Help us recognize the answers to our prayers and miracles we've received
- Encourage us to give credit and thanks where credit and thanks are due

Most of us need help in our prayer lives. It should be a great and wonderful thing, not a chore or burden. We hope to help you find that joy.

This is the day which the LORD hath made; we will rejoice and be glad in it. (Ps. 118:24)

God's Plan of Salvation for Us

~

We are God's people; He created us in His image. God loves us even though we do not follow His rules for us. Romans 3:23 lets us know this: "For all have sinned, and come short of the glory of God."

Because of the wickedness of our ways, Jesus says, "*Repent*, for the kingdom of heaven is at hand" (Matt. 4:17). *Repentance* is turning away from the things that are contrary to God; being sorry for having done those things; and turning to Jesus to be Lord of our lives.

Acts 2:38 says again "*Repent*, and be baptized everyone of you in the name of Jesus Christ for the remission of sins, and ye shall receive the gift of the Holy Spirit."

The importance of believing is stressed in Mark 16:15–16 "And he said unto them, Go ye into all the world, and preach the gospel to every creature. He that believeth and is baptized shall be saved: but he that believeth not shall be damned."

We deserved punishment: "For the wages of sin is death; but the gift of God is eternal life through Jesus Christ our Lord" (Rom. 6:23).

Because God loves us so much, He made the supreme sacrifice. He allowed His Son Jesus to become a human to fulfill the law perfectly for us, to die on the cross in our place, and to rise to glory with the Father. Romans 5:8 says, "But God commendeth his love toward us, in that, while we were yet sinners, Christ died for us."

To receive this salvation, we must believe that Jesus is God's Son and confess this with our mouths (aloud and to others) as shown in Romans 10:9–13:

> If thou shall confess with thy mouth the Lord Jesus, and shalt believe in thine heart that God hath raised him from the dead, thou shalt be saved. For with the heart man believeth unto righteousness; and with the mouth confession is made unto salvation. For the scripture saith, Whosoever believeth on him shall not be ashamed. For there is no difference between the Jew and the Greek: for the same Lord over all is rich unto all that call upon him. For whosoever shall call upon the name of the Lord shall be saved.

Pray this simple prayer and receive Jesus as your Savior:

> Dear Heavenly Father, I come to You in the name of Jesus, trusting the words of John 6:37: "Him that cometh to me I will in no wise cast out." I believe in my heart that Jesus Christ is the Son of God. I believe He was raised from the dead for my justification. I confess Him now as my Lord. Your Word says, "With the heart man believeth unto righteousness" (Rom. 10:10) and I do believe with my heart. I have now become the righteousness of God

in Christ (see 2 Cor. 5:21). And I am saved! Thank You, Lord! To You be praise and glory!

"For God so loved the world, that he gave his only begotten Son, that whosoever believeth in him should not perish, but have everlasting life" (John 3:16). This is the gospel, in a nutshell. More verification of God's love for us is found in 1 John 4:15–16:

> Whosoever shall confess that Jesus is the Son of God, God dwelleth in him, and he in God. And we have known and believed the love that God hath to us. *God is love*; and he that dwelleth in love dwelleth in God, and God in him. (Emphasis added.)

We are also strengthened by these passages in Ephesians 2:4–5:

> But God, who is rich in mercy, for his great love wherewith he loved us, Even when we were dead in sins, hath quickened us together with Christ.

We are saved by grace, as noted in Ephesians 2:8–9:

> For by *grace* are ye saved through *faith*: and that not of yourselves: it is the *gift* of God: Not of works, lest any man should boast. (Emphasis added.)

With this glorious information, we joyously say, as in Psalm 118:24, "This is [truly] the day which the LORD hath made; [I] will rejoice and be glad in it." Thank you, Lord, for inviting *me* to share in it. Amen. Hallelujah!

Prayer:
Our Gift from God

❧

Prayer is our gift from God. It is a direct route to His throne, won for us by Christ through His suffering, death, and resurrection. We must "pray without ceasing" (1 Thess. 5:17) to improve and perfect our walk with God. We must learn what to ask for and how to recognize even the smallest answers to our prayers.

Prayer is the way to receive grace and mercy, especially in time of need. This also gives us joy, to know that we are not alone against our difficulties and sorrows. Jesus Christ is there on our behalf, as written in Hebrews 4:14–16:

> Seeing then that we have a great high priest, that is passed into the heavens, Jesus the Son of God, let us hold fast our profession. For we have not a high priest which cannot be touched with the feeling of our infirmities; but was in all points tempted like as we are, yet without sin. Let us therefore come boldly unto the throne of grace,

that we may obtain mercy, and find grace to help in time of need.

John 16:24 states that prayer in Jesus' name is the way to fullness of joy: "Hitherto have ye asked nothing in my name: ask, and ye shall receive, that your joy may be full."

Prayer was a very important part of Christ's brief earthly life. Mark 1:35 says, "And in the morning, rising up a great while before day, he went out, and departed into a solitary place, and there prayed."

Jesus prays and intercedes for us constantly. It is now His main occupation. 1 Timothy 2:5 reads, "There is one God, and one mediator between God and men, the man Christ Jesus."

We pray to our heavenly Father in the name of Jesus with the help of the Holy Spirit because, as noted in Romans 8:34, "Who is he that condemneth? It is *Christ* that died, yea rather, that is risen again, who is even at the right hand of God, who also maketh intercession for us" (emphasis added). Hebrews 7:25 also confirms this.

We are each unique; none of us has the same parents, siblings, environment, friends, crises, etc. Therefore, each of us will come to God in a different way. Although we use some prayers often, like those He taught us, it is too easy to repeat them over and over without thinking about what we are saying. Our *own* words are precious and dear to the heart of God.

Praise the Lord

"For great is the LORD, and greatly to be praised" (1 Chron. 16:25). Praise and prayer should be a great and wonderful time! The Lord inhabits the praises of His people. You can be confident of His presence when you are praising Him, as shown by Psalm 22:3: "But thou art holy, O thou that inhabitest the praises of Israel."

Moment by moment let us share our joys and sorrows with Him. He is always with us. Matthew 28 ends with these comforting words: "And, lo, I am with you always, *even* unto the end of the world" (v. 20).

Revelation 5:12–13 tells us how even the angels praise our precious Lord Jesus:

> Saying with a loud voice, Worthy is the Lamb that was slain to receive power, and riches, and wisdom, and strength, and honor, and glory, and blessing. And every creature which is in heaven, and on the earth, and under the earth, and such as are in the sea, and all that are

in them, heard I saying, Blessing, and honor, and glory, and power, be unto him that sitteth upon the throne, and unto the Lamb for ever and ever.

This journal will help you feel the joy of praising Him for the wonderful things in your own life. It will help you keep in constant communication with the Lord. "This is the day which the LORD hath made; we will rejoice and be glad in it," recorded in Psalms 118:24, is a reminder that *we are special people.*

Other passages are listed under "Praise" in appendix C. Here are more references that are not listed in that section of the appendix: Psalm 33:2; Revelation 4:11; Psalm 98:1; 2 Sam. 22:4; and Psalm 100:1–4. Copy some of your *own* favorites here. Don't forget to write the reference for each verse so you can look it up again later.

FAVORITE VERSES

Make a reduced copy of your favorite hymn of praise and mount it on the next page. If you hum or sing it softly many times during the day, your subconscious mind will continue to sing praises all day long.

Sing a little of it after your evening prayer, and you will find that it stays with you all night. The Lord loves to hear us sing! Psalm 81:1–2 tells us:

Sing aloud unto God our strength: make a joyful noise unto the God of Jacob. Take a psalm and bring hither the timbrel, the pleasant harp with the psaltery.

God's desire is for us to be happy! It's good for us! "A merry heart doeth good like a medicine: but a broken spirit drieth the bones" (Prov. 17:22).

FAVORITE HYMN OF PRAISE

_____

_____

_____

_____

_____

_____

_____

_____

_____

_____

_____

_____

_____

_____

_____

_____

Pray for Forgiveness and Strength to Forgive Sin

We must, indeed, pray for forgiveness and the washing away of our sins with Jesus' blood. It is important that we *repent* to receive forgiveness from our sins. The importance of *repenting* is stated clearly in Luke 13:3, and again in v. 5. "I tell you, Nay: but, except ye *repent*, ye shall all likewise perish" (emphasis added). Also, we must pray for strength to mend our sinful ways. However, to receive forgiveness, we must also forgive others. Read Matthew 6:14–15:

> If ye forgive men their trespasses, your heavenly Father will also forgive you: But if ye forgive not men their trespasses, neither will your Father forgive your trespasses.

And again in Mark 11:25 it says, "When ye stand praying, forgive, if ye have aught against any: that your Father also which is in heaven may forgive you your trespasses."

Refer to passages in appendix C under "Forgiving Others" and "Obedience".

If we forgive and obey, then, "Being confident of this very thing, that he which hath begun a good work in you will perform it until the day of Jesus Christ" (Phil. 1:6).

Enter into His Gates with Thanksgiving

We must develop an attitude of thankfulness. "Enter into his gates with thanksgiving, and into his courts with praise: be thankful unto him, and bless his name," Psalm 100:4 tells us. Look around at the blessings He has showered upon you, and be thankful. We must be thankful even *before* we receive our blessings, not waiting until *we* recognize the blessing. He has already given us so much. Give God the glory for the things He has done for us.

Philippians 4:6–8 says:

> Be careful for nothing [don't worry]; but in every thing by prayer and supplication *with thanksgiving* let your requests be made known unto God. And the peace of God, which passeth all understanding, shall keep your hearts and minds through Christ Jesus. Finally, brethren, whatsoever things are true, whatsoever things are honest, whatsoever things are just, whatsoever things are pure, whatsoever things are lovely, whatsoever things

are of good report; if there be any virtue, and if there be any praise, think on these things. (Emphasis added.)

Glorify and praise God to prepare a thankful heart. Psalm 50:14 instructs us to "Offer unto God thanksgiving; and pay thy vows unto the most High." Show God your thankfulness with your speech, your finances, and your time.

Praying for Leaders and Those in Authority

A sequence of urgency is indicated throughout the Bible. After the praising and thanking, we will direct our attention to the first petition, as suggested in 1 Timothy 2:1–2:

> I exhort therefore, that, first of all, supplications, prayers, intercessions, and giving of thanks, be made for all men; *For kings, and for all that are in authority*; that we may lead a quiet and peaceable life in all godliness and honesty. (Emphasis added.)

We benefit by praying for wisdom for our leaders. I charge you that if every voice raised to God today were prefaced with a prayer for wise leaders and for wisdom for our leaders, we would live in a different world.

Pray for Wisdom

~

Pray for wisdom for our leaders so they can have God's help in leading a godly nation. Also, pray that God would help them make wise choices and decisions.

Pray for wisdom for yourself. It is not selfish, and it will help you in your prayer life as well as your daily life. James 1:5 notes, "If any of you lack wisdom, let him ask of God . . . and it shall be given him." It is God's will to give us the Holy Spirit to guide us in prayer, which is also wisdom.

We must be careful about criticizing our leaders. It is destructive. Ecclesiastes 10:20 points this out: "Curse not the king [or national leader], no not in thy thought; and curse not the rich in thy bedchamber: for a bird of the air [spirit being] shall carry the voice, and that which hath wings shall tell the matter." Our negative words and thoughts travel and create attitudes and situations that make things worse.

Angels, however, carry our positive thoughts and attitudes to places where they can be nurtured and grow and come true. Refer again to Philippians 4:8: "If there are any good things . . . meditate on these." This will magnify the good rather than magnify the problem. Don't concentrate on the problem.

Solomon's prayer in 1 Kings 3:1–10 includes the words: "Give therefore thy servant an understanding heart [wisdom] . . . And the speech pleased the Lord" (vv. 9–10). If we pray for wisdom, as did Solomon, for the benefit of others and ourselves, then the Lord will also be pleased with *our* prayer.

Pray in wisdom: "Ask, and it shall be given you; seek and ye shall find; knock and it shall be opened unto you." This is God's promise as recorded in Matthew 7:7.

Pray for
God's Workers

Each of us is a missionary in a sense. Our lives, our speech, and our actions tell people about our relationship with God. We are told in Matthew 5:16, "Let your light so shine before men, that they may see your good works, and glorify your Father which is in heaven."

Each of us has an obligation to pray for those who are training to become missionaries, pastors, and teachers. Our financial help is also needed to help them finish school and get started in the field, reaching people for Jesus. They *are* our ministry.

The wheat tends to see only the wheat, and the chaff sees only the chaff. *Help us to see the good in people, Lord, so that we may be counted among the wheat. Amen.*

Praying for Others

~

God wants the saints to join Him in bringing others under the blood of the Lamb. He could do it alone, but it is His plan for us also to intercede for them. These prayers are near to His heart. Our commission is stated in 2 Corinthians 5:20:

> Now then we are ambassadors for Christ, as though God did beseech you by us: we pray you in Christ's stead, be ye reconciled to God.

Also, "Being confident of this very thing, that he which hath begun a good work in you will perform it until the day of Jesus Christ" (Phil. 1:6).

We should pray for others' health and well being. Immersing ourselves in these prayers will bring about the joy and healing we need in *our own* lives.

1 Corinthians 13:8 tells us that "[Love] never faileth." Verse 13 reassures us, "And now abideth faith, hope, charity, these three; but the greatest of these is charity [love]." You see, faith gets you started, but it always leads to mountains! Hope keeps you going. Pray that the Lord will lead you to the person to whom He wants to speak through your life today. Love makes it beautiful. The greatest of these is love.

"Confess your faults one to another, and pray for one another, that ye may be healed" (James 5:16). *Healed* in that your need may be healed, that you may receive the answer to your prayer.

Peter urges us to be ever mindful of the needs of others: "Finally, be ye all of one mind, having compassion one of another, love as brethren, be pitiful, be courteous" (1 Pet. 3:8). When we help and pray for others, God gives us this promise in John 13:27: "Peace I leave with you, my peace I give unto you: not as the world giveth, give I unto you."

If we seek God's blessings for others, especially His spiritual blessings, we will also receive His blessings. We see this in Matthew 6:33:

> But seek ye first the kingdom of God, and his righteousness; and all these things shall be added unto you.

Petitions for Ourselves

O f ourselves, we don't know what to pray for, but Romans 8:26–27 states,

> Likewise the Spirit also helpeth our infirmities: for we know not what we should pray for as we ought: but the *Spirit* itself maketh intercession for us with groanings which cannot be uttered. And he that searcheth the hearts knoweth what is the mind of the Spirit, because he maketh intercession for the saints *according to the will of God.* (Emphasis added.)

But God is quick to tell us how to pray in the will of God: "If any of you lack wisdom, let him ask of God, that giveth to all men liberally, and upbraideth not; and it *shall* be given him" (James 1:5, emphasis added). So when we ask for wisdom, we know we will receive it.

We also know that when we pray for the Holy Spirit, we will receive Him. "If ye then, being evil, know how to give good gifts unto your children: how much more *shall* your heavenly Father give the Holy Spirit to them that ask him?" (Luke 11:13, emphasis added).

With wisdom and the Holy Spirit to guide us into the will of God, we can know that we *are*, therefore, in the will of God. John shares:

> And this is the confidence that we have in him, that, if we ask any thing according to his will, he heareth us: And if we know that he hear us, whatsoever we ask, we know that we have the petitions that we desired of him. (1 John 5:14–15)

Therefore, we must pray for things in the name of Jesus, in the will of God, for the glory of God, and *with faith and confidence in God.*

> Whatsoever ye shall ask *in my name*, that will I do, that the *Father may be glorified in the Son.* If ye shall ask any thing *in my name*, I will do it. (John 14:13–14, emphasis added)

Ask and pray with faith. God's Word says:

> Therefore I say unto you, What things soever ye desire, when ye pray, believe that ye receive them, and ye shall have them. (Mark 11:24)

> So then faith *cometh* by hearing, and hearing by the word of God. (Rom. 10:17)

> If ye abide in me, and my words abide in you, ye shall ask what ye will, and it shall be done unto you. (John 15:7)

Prayer can be hindered in several ways. Examine yourself to see if any of the following apply to your life.

1. **Selfish prayers**.

   Ye ask, and receive not, because ye ask amiss, that ye may consume it upon your lusts. (James 4:3)

2. **Continued sin**. Repent and ask forgiveness.

   And whatsoever we ask, we receive of him, because we keep his commandments, and do those things that are pleasing in his sight. (1 John 3:22)

   If I regard iniquity in my heart, the Lord will not hear me. (Ps. 66:18)

   Behold, the Lord's hand is not shortened, that it cannot save; neither his ear heavy, that it cannot hear: But your iniquities have separated between you and your God, and your sins have hid his face from you, that he will not hear. (Isa. 59:1–2)

3. **Lack of generosity to God's work, to the poor, etc.**

   Give, and it shall be given unto you; good measure, pressed down, and shaken together, and running over, shall men give into your bosom. For with the same measure that ye mete withal [give out] it shall be measured to you again. (Luke 6:38)

   But my God shall supply all your need according to his riches in glory by Christ Jesus. (Phil. 4:19)

4. **An unforgiving attitude in relationships**.

   And when ye stand praying, forgive, if ye have ought against any: that your Father also which is in heaven may forgive you your trespasses. (Mark 11:25)

   Likewise, ye husbands, dwell with them according to knowledge, giving honour unto the wife, as unto the weaker vessel, and as being *heirs together* of the grace of life; that your prayers be not hindered. (1 Pet. 3:7, emphasis added)

5. **Idols in the heart** (objects of our affection put before God). Those who love their business, reputation, family, husbands, wife, children, grandchildren, money, and possessions more than they love God— should they receive answers to prayer?

   Son of man, these men have set up their idols in their heart, and put the stumbling block of their iniquity before their face; should I be inquired of at all by them? (Ezek. 14:3)

6. **Firmly believe**. Have faith that the answer to your prayers will come. Have confidence in God.

   But my God shall supply all your need according to his riches in glory by Christ Jesus. (Phil. 4:19)

   Cast not away therefore your confidence, which hath great recompence of reward. (Heb. 10:35)

Let Us Have Confidence

~

The Bible tells us, "But my God shall supply all your need according to his riches in glory by Christ Jesus" (Phil. 4:19), and, "Let us therefore come boldly unto the throne of grace, that we may obtain mercy, and find grace to help in time of need" (Heb. 4:16). This last passage encourages us to have confidence that the Lord can and will supply our needs and answer our prayers. More encouragement is found in the following passages:

> And this is the confidence that we have in him, that, if we ask any thing according to his will, he heareth us: And if we know that he hear us, whatsoever we ask, we know that we _have_ the petitions that we desired of him. (1 John 5:14–15, emphasis added)

> For the Lord shall be thy confidence, and shall keep thy foot from being taken. (Prov. 3:26)

I can do all things through Christ which strengtheneth me. (Phil. 4:13)

Cast not away therefore your confidence, which hath great recompence of reward. For we have need of patience, that, after ye have done the will of God, ye might receive the promise. (Heb. 10:35–36)

Nay, in all these things we are *more* than conquerors through him that loved us. (Rom. 8:37, emphasis added)

Being confident of this very thing, that he which hath begun a good work in you will perform it until the day of Jesus Christ. (Phil. 1:6)

In whom we have boldness and access with confidence by the faith of him. (Eph. 3:12)

Waiting on the Lord

Prayer is not just asking for things, it is *giving God time and attention* to communicate with us. Give him the time to help solve our daily problems. Wait on the Lord—alone and uninterrupted.

This is a time to be spiritually alert and watchful that our prayers are not shallow and selfish, a time to ask the Holy Spirit how to pray and how to receive the answers to our prayer. Prayer in the Spirit is most powerful.

By focusing on God's love for us, with undivided attention, we can absorb divine instructions from God for our daily lives. God does answer prayer, sometimes in an hour, sometimes in many years. We must wait—*for* Him and *on* Him—and believe.

The promise to those who wait for the Lord's direction in their lives is found in Isaiah 40:31:

> But they that wait upon the Lord shall renew *their* strength; they shall mount up with wings as eagles; they shall run, and not be weary; *and* they shall walk, and not faint.

Answers to Prayer

To receive, we must pray in the name of Jesus, who has bought us with His precious blood and to whom we belong. We are His inheritance. The whole chapter of John 17 tells us in many ways who we are and how precious we are. John 14 tells us:

> Whatsoever ye shall ask *in my name*, that will I do, that the *Father may be glorified* in the Son. If ye shall ask any thing *in my name*, I will do it. (vv. 13–14, emphasis added)

To receive, we must pray according to His will, as instructed in 1 John 5:14–15:

> And this is the confidence that we have in him, that, if we ask any thing according to his will, he heareth us: And if we know that he hear us, whatsoever we ask, we know that we have the petitions that we desired of him.

To know that we are praying in His will, review the scriptures quoted in appendix C.

Remember to thank God for all the gifts He has given. Many of us are so quick to prompt a child by reminding, "What do you say, now?" that the child doesn't even have a chance to show if he would remember to say "thank you" by himself or not. Yet sometimes we ourselves brush by gift after gift, miracle after miracle, without noticing or acknowledging them. We refuse to call the small, everyday blessings "miracles," believing that a miracle has to be an earthshaking event in order to qualify. This small blessing removed, however, would take a "miracle" to mend the situation that developed as a result of the absence of that blessing. I ask you, then, was that blessing a miracle?

Many of us pray for—and receive—little blessings, but when they quietly happen, we forget that we asked for them. God never says, "What do you say, now?" He just gives and gives and gives. As adult "children of God," *we* have to remind *ourselves*, because we don't want to be like ungrateful children.

The purpose of this journal is to help us remember! Use it! Write your prayer notes! Write down the answers as they come. Keep track of the big things *and* the little things. Watch for and recognize your miracles! Resolve to use this book every day, and soon you will realize how blessed you really are.

To remember the answers to prayers and special blessings is to edify ourselves and others by sharing what the Lord has done in our lives. It is often not enough to relate a blessing without noting the touch of the Lord. Another person may not receive the insight without a small explanation. By sharing, we both can be edified.

This journal is divided into areas for prayer requests, leaving room to note answers beside the requests. A record of "walking with God" will serve to edify yourself when you are feeling down. Read what you have written.

In times of feeling down, we often cannot recall the good things God has done for us. But going back and reading these answers to prayer will lift our spirits. Entering these gifts into the journal will provide a place to go when depressed.

We must learn to recognize the little joys that "just turn out right" even before we knew we needed them and made a request for them. Thank the Lord. Make a note of these joys in your journal. These same joys will edify you later.

Answers to prayers come in many ways. Perhaps God will change the circumstances to accommodate the problem. Perhaps He will change the problem itself—in a better way than you had thought of. Perhaps He will change your heart and give you wisdom to cope. Or perhaps, He will use the struggle to strengthen you for a future confrontation with difficulty or temptation.

Because we have turned the rudder, God will turn the ship. God moves through prayer.

Praises to Close Our Time of Prayer

∼

This is the day which the LORD hath made; we will rejoice and be glad in it. (Ps. 118:24)

For this day is holy unto our Lord: neither be ye sorry; for the joy of the LORD is your strength. (Neh. 8:10)

I will bless the LORD at all times: his praise shall continually be in my mouth. (Ps. 34:1)

If you have another favorite hymn, write or paste it here.

_____

_____

_____

_____

_____

_____

Prayer in Time of Oppression and Depression

One successful way to deal with any oppressive situation—whether health, heartache, financial, or whatever —is to enter into intercessory prayer for others, especially for someone who is really in need of your prayers. Forget about yourself, and become totally concerned with the salvation and well being of someone else. Refer to chapter 9 for help in getting started.

> The LORD also will be a refuge for the oppressed, a refuge in times of trouble. And they that know thy name will put their trust in thee: for thou, LORD, hath not forsaken them that seek thee. (Ps. 9:9–10)

Here is a short prayer that has helped many:

> Dear Father, Help me to learn quickly the lesson that this situation is to teach me. Help me to deal wisely, to

bring a speedy and lasting solution. In Jesus' name, I ask. Amen.

This more comprehensive prayer may be used also:

Dear Lord, I am distressed. Grant me wisdom to find the pathway through this difficult time. You have said in Isaiah 41:10, "Fear thou not; for I am with thee." Guide me in my decisions to comply with Your will. Protect me from the evil that would harm me and lead me astray. Psalm 23 says that we should fear no evil. Teach me quickly, Lord, the things I should learn from this situation, that I may be relieved of this burden and get on with the new challenges You have for me. Give me the strength to overcome as You have promised in Galatians 6:9: "And let us not be weary in well doing: for in due season we shall reap, if we faint not." Lord, deliver me from this oppression as promised in Psalm 50:15 where You say, "And call upon me in the day of trouble: I will deliver thee, and thou shalt glorify me." Grant me Your peace, in Jesus' name. Amen.

Forgive yourself! God has already forgiven you if you have repented. He remembers your sins no more! Don't continue to punish yourself for sins that God has already forgiven and forgotten, as shown in these passages:

For I will be merciful to their unrighteousness, and their sins and their iniquities will I remember no more. (Heb. 8:12)

And their sins and iniquities will I remember no more. (Heb. 10:17)

And they shall teach no more every man his neighbour, and every man his brother, saying, Know the LORD: for they shall all know me, from the least of them unto the greatest of them, saith the LORD: for I will forgive their iniquity, and I will remember their sin no more. (Jer. 31:34)

The secret is that we *must bury the past*. Philippians 3:13–14 says:

Brethren, I count not myself to have apprehended: but this one thing I do, forgetting those things which are behind, and reaching forth unto those things which are before, I press toward the mark for the prize of the high calling of God in Christ Jesus.

This includes burdensome guilt and haunting memories. Remember 2 Corinthians 5:17: "Therefore if any man be in Christ, he is a new creature: old things are passed away; behold, all things are become new." This is good news, indeed!

Also, take heart from Isaiah 40:29–31:

He giveth power to the faint . . . the youths shall faint and be weary, and the young men shall utterly fail: But they that wait upon the LORD shall renew their strength; they shall mount up with wings as eagles; they shall run, and not be weary; and they shall walk, and not faint.

Other passages for your consideration are: Luke 18:1; 2 Chronicles 1:7–11; Proverbs 3:24; Psalm 4:5.

You will also receive comfort from Psalm 91. It is so encouraging, I have included it here in its entirety.

He that dwelleth in the secret place of the most High shall abide under the shadow of the Almighty. I will say of the LORD, he is my refuge and my fortress: my God; in him will I trust. Surely he shall deliver thee from the snare of the fowler, and from the noisome pestilence. He shall cover thee with his feathers, and under his wings shalt thou trust: his truth shall be thy shield and buckler [armor]. Thou shalt not be afraid for the terror by night; nor for the arrow that flieth by day. Nor for the pestilence that walketh in darkness; nor for the destruction that wasteth at noonday. A thousand shall fall at thy side, and ten thousand at thy right hand; but it shall not come nigh thee. Only with thine eyes shalt thou behold and see the reward of the wicked. Because thou hast made the LORD, which is my refuge, even the most High, thy habitation. There shall no evil befall thee, neither shall any plague come nigh thy dwelling. For he shall give his angels charge over thee, to keep thee in all thy ways. They shall bear thee up in their hands, lest thou dash thy foot against a stone. Thou shall tread upon the lion and adder; the young lion and the dragon shall thou trample under feet. Because he hath set his love upon me, therefore will I deliver him; I will set him on high, because he hath known my name. He shall call upon me, and I will answer him: I will be with him in trouble; I will deliver him, and honor him. With long life will I satisfy him, and shew him my salvation.

The Power of Cumulative Prayer

~

In a Buddhist temple, in the city of Rangoon, hangs the largest and most beautiful bell in the East. But it was not always there. Indeed not! It had been hidden beneath the surface of a river during the Angle-Burman wars. Its great weight had caused it to settle deep into the silt and muck of the river's bottom. All efforts by many engineers failed to rescue the bell.

Finally, a humble priest asked permission to try to retrieve it, with the condition that the bell be given to his temple if his rescue attempts were successful.

This agreed, he and his helpers gathered huge amounts of bamboo rods. The buoyancy of these rods makes it difficult to hold more than one or two down under the water, and so it was that divers took the rods down, one at a time, and fastened them securely to the bottom of the bell. After many thousand rods had been taken down and the situation began to look hopeless, someone noticed that the bell had begun to move a little.

With renewed vigor, more rods were gathered and fastened to the bell. Soon it rose, with dignity, to the surface. It was the effort of the humble people, a little at a time, working together, that accomplished this great deed.

So it is with prayer. God says, "Where two or three are gathered together in my name, there am I in the midst of them" (Matt. 18:20). In James 5:15 we find,

> And the prayer of faith shall save the sick, and the Lord shall raise him up; and if he have committed sins, they shall be forgiven him.

The above verse in James is preceded by these words: "Is any sick among you? let him call for the elders of the church; and let them pray over him, anointing him with oil in the name of the Lord" (James 5:14).

It is my firm belief that a concerted cumulative offering of prayer by more of us "little people," along with those of our spiritual leaders, would change the character of leaders all around the world. God is moved by our prayers. He hears; He listens; He answers the prayers of His own.

Gather for intercessory prayers against the immoral conditions of government, society, television, and ourselves. If we want them to be changed, they will be changed. God has promised *Whatsoever!*

And let us not forget our own hearts. We must continue to ask that our hearts will be changed into alignment with the will of the Lord. Then we will be ready for new challenges.

Did not God tell us:

> Ye are the light of the world. A city that is set on a hill cannot be hid. Neither do men light a candle, and put it under a bushel, but on a candlestick; and it giveth light unto all that are in the house. Let your light so shine before men, that they may see your good works, and glorify your Father which is in heaven. (Matt 5:14–16)?

Praying and Meditating in the Scriptures

〜

While reading the Scriptures, oftentimes a passage will jump out at you with a special meaning. It will speak directly to your needs. When you discover these verses, claim them for your own. Stop and quietly meditate on them. Ponder their every aspect; receive those truths into your heart.

Copy the verses and references into your journal in appendix C. Or copy them into your current prayer.

Quote this special scripture to God in your prayer. He loves to have us review His promises with Him. When we ask for the Spirit of God to pray in us, He does so according to the will of God. That heavy sigh that comes from the heart? God knows what it says.

Praying When We Don't Feel Like Praying

~

What should we do when we don't feel like praying? What if your heart feels like a cold lump of stone? Rejoice! There is blessed help. Come quietly to the Lord and tell Him how cold and prayerless your heart feels. Ask for the Holy Spirit to warm your heart and draw you near in prayer and love. Be truthful with God; He knows your heart.

Luke 11:13 tells us,

> If ye then, being evil, know how to give good gifts unto your children: how much more shall your heavenly Father give the *Holy Spirit* to them that ask him? (Emphasis added.)

Romans 8:26–27 encourages us further:

> Likewise the Spirit also helpeth our infirmities: for we know not what we should pray for as we ought: but the

Spirit itself maketh intercession for us with groanings which cannot be uttered. And he that searcheth the hearts knoweth what is the mind of the Spirit, because he maketh intercession for the saints according to the will of God.

God understands the sigh that comes from a heavy heart.

Don't get impatient with the Lord. He will answer your prayers "in due season" (see Gal. 6:9). Isaiah 40:31 says,

But they that wait upon the LORD shall renew *their* strength; they shall mount up with wings as eagles; they shall run, and not be weary; *and* they shall walk, and not faint.

Never give up on anyone or anything. Miracles happen all the time! Keeping this journal is designed to help you *through* these times. Page through the prayers you have recorded. Check out the answers. Note the times you have been blessed—before you had even asked. Never neglect to include these things in your journal text; they are there to edify you in times like these. Reviewing precious times with your Lord will draw you near to Him again.

Psalm 9:9 reminds us that "The LORD also will be a refuge for the oppressed, a refuge in times of trouble."

Giving to Receive

~

G od loveth a cheerful giver" (2 Cor. 9:7). And He will not be outdone. An incident in my own life may not compare with happenings in others' lives, but it serves to illustrate this truth.

I had just written a check to one of the Lord's ministries and had placed it on the dining room table, ready to mail. A knock came at the door, and a lady asked about some things I had for sale. I didn't know this lady, but she had heard about my work. I really needed to make that sale, and the Lord was right there. She came in and bought four times as much value as the amount of the check I had written. What continues to amaze me is that I hadn't even mailed the check yet.

Of course, not every gift will be "refunded" within a few minutes, or hours, or days. But God will provide and return your blessing. We should never give, however, to get something. God sees into our hearts and knows our motives.

The writer of Genesis had this to say about seedtime and harvest, giving and receiving: "While the earth remaineth, seedtime and harvest, and cold and heat, and summer and winter, and day and night shall not cease" (v. 8:22).

God also says in Malachi 3:10:

> Bring ye all the tithes into the storehouse, that there may be meat in mine house, and prove me now herewith, saith the LORD of hosts, if I will not open you the windows of heaven, and pour you out a blessing, that there shall not be room enough to receive it.

"Love gifts" are gifts of time, prayers, material things—new or keepsakes—that we can give or share. We don't have to give all our keepsakes away, but we can share the memories behind them. In appendix A is a special page for recording love gifts received, already given, or yet to give or make for someone.

Witnessing to Others

Witnessing about what the Lord is doing and has done in our lives is a very necessary part of prayer life. After our prayer, after our miracle, we should testify to our children about the blessings and miracles God has done for us. This is especially meaningful if done by *fathers*. In Joshua 4:21–23, God stresses the importance of *fathers* testifying to the children.

Witnessing to our children and our friends will help them identify their miracles and will strengthen their faith. We should be careful not to offend others when witnessing. James warns us to bridle the tongue (see James 1:26) and speak in line with the Word. We must lead, not dictate.

Sharing spiritual gifts and experiences creates the spiritual bond we need to help us in our spiritual warfare. We all need that moral and spiritual support at times. By having the information available in this journal, we can refer to it for our own edification. It will help us soar over our problems, knowing God will support us and bring us to a better place.

When we have accepted our healing, yet all the symptoms are still there, what do we say when asked, "How are you?" Those of us of faith might share our healing experience. For others, it would be appropriate to say, "I believe that I am getting better," or, "I feel that I am improving." We shouldn't, however, recount all the symptoms that haven't left us yet.

Romans 10:10 says, "For with the heart man believeth unto righteousness; and with the mouth confession is made unto salvation." By repeating the good things or the bad things that may happen, we truly bring them to pass. Keeping track of joys, accomplishments, and goals, however, will help bring them to fruition.

Using This Journal

~~

This journal is intended to help guide you in your prayer life. Because the Lord loves to have us quote His Word to Him, I have included many promises for you. References are made to the different pages in the text to review as you outline your prayers in your own words.

The many repetitions could not be helped. Everything cannot be said at once; thus referring back to some of the same information is necessary. By reading these passages over and over, you will soon commit them to memory for use in witnessing to others.

After reading through the text, make the journal your own by copying your favorite hymn of praise on your designated page. Make it your theme song, and hum it often throughout the day. Copy your favorite praise passages on the same page, along with their references.

Then continue on to each section, filling in your own words and thoughts. I've included room, in the area for prayer requests, for answers to be noted beside them. Refer each time to the original chapter for help in designing your own petitions.

When you have used the same prayer for a short time, you will want to revise and add to it. Although, at first, there is room for added notes on the original pages, you will soon want to move into the next section of the journal. Remember to bring forward the major answers to prayers so that you will be reminded to give thanks for them. Review the old prayers and thoughts often.

Pray about everything. Even one sentence directed toward God, acknowledges your constant communication with Him. Prayers don't have to be long and drawn out.

Before you begin your prayer, take a few moments here to make some notes. Thinking back over the recent days, list blessings you have received. Also list friends who need your prayerful support. Come back later and make a note of the solution.

Using this prayer journal faithfully will help you receive the benefit of this promise from Job 22:21: "Acquaint now thyself with him, and be at peace: thereby good shall come unto thee."

1. Recent blessings remembered with praise and thanksgiving:

   _____

   _____

2. Special people on my prayer list: _____

   _____

   _____

3. Answers to prayers noted: _____

   _____

   _____

Personal Prayers

D ear Heavenly Father,   We come to You in the name of Jesus, Your only Son and our Lord. We praise and thank You for sending Him to atone for our sin. For this we are forever grateful. We thank You for your love and grace in sending Him.

Now continue with your praise section of your prayer, as noted:

- In the PRAISE section on page 19
- FORGIVENESS on page 23
- THANKSGIVING on page 25
- LEADERS (write specific names) on page 27
- WISDOM on page 29
- GOD'S WORKERS AND OTHERS on pages 31 and 33
- OURSELVES on page 35
- CLOSING PRAISES on page 152

Dear Heavenly Father, We come in the name of Jesus with praise and thanksgiving. (Now add your own prayer)

These pages are for your personal prayers:

Prayer Requests: *Answers Noted:*

Prayer Requests: Answers Noted:

Prayer Requests: *Answers Noted:*

Prayer Requests: *Answers Noted:*

Prayer Requests: *Answers Noted:*

Prayer Requests: *Answers Noted:*

Prayer Requests: *Answers Noted:*

Prayer Requests: *Answers Noted:*

Prayer Requests: Answers Noted:

Prayer Requests: *Answers Noted:*

Prayer Requests: *Answers Noted:*

Prayer Requests: *Answers Noted:*

Prayer Requests: Answers Noted:

Prayer Requests: *Answers Noted:*

Prayer Requests: *Answers Noted:*

Prayer Requests: *Answers Noted:*

Prayer Requests: *Answers Noted:*

Prayer Requests: *Answers Noted:*

Prayer Requests: *Answers Noted:*

Prayer Requests: *Answers Noted:*

Prayer Requests: *Answers Noted:*

Prayer Requests: Answers Noted:

Prayer Requests: Answers Noted:

Prayer Requests: *Answers Noted:*

Prayer Requests: *Answers Noted:*

Prayer Requests: *Answers Noted:*

Prayer Requests: *Answers Noted:*

Prayer Requests: *Answers Noted:*

Prayer Requests: *Answers Noted:*

Prayer Requests: *Answers Noted:*

Prayer Requests:

Answers Noted:

Prayer Requests: *Answers Noted:*

Prayer Requests: *Answers Noted:*

Prayer Requests: *Answers Noted:*

Prayer Requests: *Answers Noted:*

Prayer Requests: *Answers Noted:*

Prayer Requests:

Answers Noted:

Prayer Requests: *Answers Noted:*

Prayer Requests: *Answers Noted:*

Prayer Requests: *Answers Noted:*

Prayer Requests:

Answers Noted:

Prayer Requests: Answers Noted:

Prayer Requests: *Answers Noted:*

Prayer Requests: Answers Noted:

Prayer Requests: *Answers Noted:*

Prayer Requests: *Answers Noted:*

Prayer Requests: *Answers Noted:*

Prayer Requests: Answers Noted:

Prayer Requests: *Answers Noted:*

Prayer Requests: *Answers Noted:*

Prayer Requests: *Answers Noted:*

Prayer Requests: Answers Noted:

Prayer Requests: *Answers Noted:*

Prayer Requests: *Answers Noted:*

Prayer Requests: *Answers Noted:*

Prayer Requests: *Answers Noted:*

Prayer Requests: *Answers Noted:*

Prayer Requests: *Answers Noted:*

Prayer Requests: *Answers Noted:*

Prayer Requests: Answers Noted:

Prayer Requests: *Answers Noted:*

Prayer Requests: *Answers Noted:*

Prayer Requests: *Answers Noted:*

Prayer Requests: Answers Noted:

Prayer Requests: *Answers Noted:*

Prayer Requests: *Answers Noted:*

Prayer Requests: *Answers Noted:*

Prayer Requests: *Answers Noted:*

Prayer Requests: *Answers Noted:*

Prayer Requests: Answers Noted:

Prayer Requests: *Answers Noted:*

Prayer Requests: *Answers Noted:*

Prayer Requests: *Answers Noted:*

Prayer Requests: *Answers Noted:*

Prayer Requests: *Answers Noted:*

Prayer Requests: Answers Noted:

Prayer Requests: *Answers Noted:*

Prayer Requests: *Answers Noted:*

Prayer Requests: *Answers Noted:*

Love Gifts

This special page for recording "love gifts" is to help you remember to share your talents and special gifts. Use this time to reflect on friends and acquaintances, to understand and appreciate them. By recording our intentions here, we can avoid the forgetfulness that often happens after a fleeting thought. Reviewing this may be a reminder for a gift or prayer to bring that special blessing.

LOVE GIFTS THAT I HAVE RECEIVED:	LOVE GIFTS I HAVE GIVEN TO UPLIFT SOMEONE'S SPIRIT:	LOVE GIFTS YET TO MAKE FOR:

Revelation 1:9-19

Following is a written picture of our glorified Savior who is coming again for all His saints. This is the vision of Jesus as recorded in Revelation:

I John, who also am your brother, and companion in tribulation, and in the kingdom and patience of Jesus Christ, was in the isle that is called Patmos, for the word of God, and for the testimony of Jesus Christ. I was in the Spirit on the Lord's day, and heard behind me a great voice, as of a trumpet, Saying, I am Alpha and Omega, the first and the last: and, What thou seest, write in a book, and send it unto the seven churches which are in Asia; unto Ephesus, and unto Smyrna, and unto Pergamos, and unto Thyatira, and unto Sardis, and unto Philadelphia, and unto Laodicea. And I turned to see the voice that spake with me. And being turned, I saw seven golden candlesticks; And in the midst of the seven candlesticks, one like unto the Son of man, clothed with a garment down to the foot, and girt about the paps with a golden girdle. His head and his hairs were white like wool, as white as snow; and his eyes were as a flame of fire; And his feet like unto fine brass, as if they burned in a furnace; and his voice as the sound of many waters. And he had in his right hand seven stars: and out of his mouth went a sharp two-edged sword; and his countenance was as the sun shineth in his strength. And when I saw him, I fell at his feet as dead. And he laid his right hand upon me, saying unto me, Fear not; I am the first and the last: I am he that liveth, and was dead; and, behold, I am alive for evermore, Amen; and have the keys of hell and of death. Write the things which thou hast seen, and the things which are, and the things which shall be hereafter.

This is the powerful, glorified Jesus who intercedes for us.

Selected Favorite Passages

~

These special passages are listed here to edify and strengthen you in your prayer life. Use these as a starting place. Add your own and others as they are revealed to you. Some space has been left for you to write yours in this list, besides writing them within your prayers. Blessings!

FINDING THE WILL OF GOD

If any of you lack wisdom, let him ask of God, that giveth to all men liberally, and upbraideth not; and it shall be given him. (James 1:5)

Thy word is a lamp unto my feet, and a light unto my path. (Ps. 119:105)

For this God is our God for ever and ever; he will be our guide even unto death. (Ps. 48:14)

Be careful for nothing, but in every thing by prayer and supplication with thanksgiving let your requests be made known unto God. And the peace of God, which passes all understanding, shall keep your hearts and minds through Christ Jesus. Finally, my brethren, whatsoever things are true, whatsoever things are honest, whatsoever things are just, whatsoever things are pure, whatsoever things are lovely, whatsoever things are of good report; if there be any virtue, and if there be any praise, think on these things. (Phil. 4:6–8)

PRAISE

Bless the LORD, O my soul: and all that is within me, *bless* his holy name. Bless the LORD, O my soul, and forget not all his benefits: Who forgiveth all thine iniquities; who healeth all thy diseases; Who redeemeth thy life from destruction; who crowneth thee with lovingkindness and tender mercies; Who satisfieth thy mouth with good things; so that thy youth is renewed like the eagle's. (Ps. 103:1–5)

But thou, O LORD, art a shield for me; my glory and the lifter up of mine head. (Ps. 3:3)

And I give unto them eternal life; and they shall never perish, neither shall any man pluck them out of my hand. (John 10:28)

I will call on the LORD, who is worthy to be praised: so shall I be saved from mine enemies. (2 Sam. 22:4)

Whoso offereth praise, glorifieth me: and to him that ordereth his conversation aright will I shew the salvation of God. (Ps. 50:23)

O Lord, thou art my God; I will exalt thee, I will praise thy name; for thou hast done wonderful things; thy counsels of old are faithfulness and truth. (Isa. 25:1)

With men [it] is impossible; but with God all things are possible. (Matt. 19:26)

God, who is rich in mercy, for his great love wherewith he loved us . . . hath quickened us together with Christ . . . and made us sit together in heavenly places in Christ Jesus. (Eph. 2:4–6)

Now the God of hope fill you with all joy and peace in believing, that ye may abound in hope, through the power of the Holy Ghost. (Rom. 15:13)

Faith and Believing

Again I say unto you, That if two of you shall agree on earth as touching any thing that they shall ask, it shall be done for them of my Father which is in heaven. For where two or three are gathered together in my name, there am I in the midst of them. (Matt. 18:19–20)

And they were all filled with the Holy Ghost, and began to speak with other tongues, as the Spirit gave them utterance. (Acts 2:4)

Let us therefore come boldly unto the throne of grace, that we may obtain mercy, and find grace to help in time of need. (Heb. 4:16)

For God so loved the world, that he gave his only begotten Son, that whosoever believeth in him should not perish, but have everlasting life. (John 3:16)

For I will restore health unto thee, and I will heal thee of thy wounds, saith the LORD. (Jer. 30:17)

If ye had faith as a grain of mustard seed, ye might say unto this sycamine tree, Be thou plucked up by the root, and be thou planted in the sea: and it should obey you. (Luke 17:6)

Jesus said unto him, If thou canst believe, all things are possible to him that believeth. (Mark 9:23)

For with the heart man believeth unto righteousness; and with the mouth confession is made unto salvation. (Rom. 10:10)

OBEDIENCE

What? know ye not that your body is the temple of the Holy Ghost which is in you, which ye have of God, and ye are not your own? (1 Cor. 6:19)

If any man among you seem to be religious, and bridleth not his tongue, but deceiveth his own heart, this man's religion is vain. (James 1:26)

A new commandment I give unto you, That ye love one another; as I have loved you, that ye also love one another. By this shall all men know that ye are my disciple; if ye have love one to another. (John 13:34–35)

Watch and pray, that ye enter not into temptation: the spirit indeed is willing, but the flesh is weak. (Matt. 26:41)

But the fruit of the Spirit is love, joy, peace, longsuffering, gentleness, goodness, faith, meekness, temperance: against such there is no law. (Gal. 5:22–23)

COURAGE AND INNER STRENGTH

Beloved, think it not strange concerning the fiery trial which is to try you, as though some strange thing happened unto you: But rejoice, inasmuch as ye are partakers of Christ's sufferings; that, when his glory shall be revealed, ye may be glad also with exceeding joy. (1 Pet. 4:12–13)

For I am persuaded, that neither death, nor life, nor angels, nor principalities, nor powers, nor things present, nor things to come, Nor height, nor depth, nor any other creature, shall be able to separate us from the love of God, which is in Christ Jesus our Lord. (Rom. 8:38–39)

I can do all things through Christ which strengtheneth me. (Phil. 4:13)

Being confident of this very thing, that he which hath begun a good work in you will perform it until the day of Jesus Christ. (Phil. 1:6)

Be sober, be vigilant; because your adversary the devil, as a roaring lion, walketh about, seeking whom he may devour: Whom resist stedfast in the faith. (1 Pet. 5:8–9)

Submit yourselves therefore to God. Resist the devil, and he will flee from you. (James 4:7)

But if any provide not for his own, and specially for those of his own house, he hath denied the faith, and is worse than an infidel. (1 Tim. 5:8)

Train up a child in the way he should go; and when he is old, he will not depart from it. (Prov. 22:6)

For thou art my lamp, O LORD: and the LORD will lighten my darkness. (2 Sam. 22:29)

God is my strength and power: and he maketh my way perfect. (2 Sam. 22:33)

For God hath not given us the spirit of fear; but of power, and of love, and of a sound mind. (2 Tim. 1:7)

But my God shall supply all your need according to his riches in glory by Christ Jesus. (Phil. 4:19)

FORGIVING OTHERS

For if ye forgive men their trespasses, your heavenly Father will also forgive you: But if ye forgive not men their trespasses, neither will your Father forgive your trespasses. (Matt. 6:14–15)

Take heed to yourselves: If thy brother trespass against thee, rebuke him; and if he repent, forgive him. (Luke 17:3)

And when ye stand praying, forgive, if ye have ought against any: that your Father also which is in heaven may forgive you your trespasses. (Mark 11:25)

If we confess our sins, he is faithful and just to forgive us our sins, and to cleanse us from all unrighteousness. (1 John 1:9)

IN THE NAME OF JESUS

For there is one God, and one mediator between God and men, the man Christ Jesus. (1 Tim. 2:5)

Behold, I stand at the door, and knock: if any man hear my voice, and open the door, I will come in to him, and will sup with him, and he with me. (Rev. 3:20)

For ye have not received the spirit of bondage again to fear; but ye have received the Spirit of adoption, whereby we cry, Abba, Father. (Rom. 8:15)

I am the door: by me if any man enter in, he shall be saved, and shall go in and out, and find pasture. (John 10:9)

Keep yourselves in the love of God, looking for the mercy of our Lord Jesus Christ unto eternal life. (Jude 21)

God hath given to us eternal life, and this life is in his son. He that hath the Son hath life. (1 John 5:11–12)

Verily, verily, I say unto you, Whatsoever ye shall ask the Father, in my name, he will give it you. (John 16:23)

GIVING AND RECEIVING

Give, and it shall be given unto you; good measure, pressed down, and shaken together, and running over, shall men give into your bosom. For with the same measure that ye mete withal it shall be measured to you again. (Luke 6:38)

Bring ye all the tithes into the storehouse, that there may be meat in mine house, and prove me now herewith, saith the LORD of hosts, if I will not open you the windows of heaven, and pour you out a blessing that there shall not be room enough to receive it. (Mal. 3:10)

A good man leaveth an inheritance to his children's children: and the wealth of the sinner is laid up for the just. (Prov. 13:22)

Beloved, I wish above all things that thou mayest prosper and be in health, even as thy soul prospereth. (3 John 2)

And it shall come to pass, that before they call, I will answer; and while they are yet speaking, I will hear. (Isa. 65:24)

Every good gift and every perfect gift is from above, and cometh down from the Father of lights, with whom is no variableness, neither shadow of turning. (James 1:17)

While the earth remaineth, seedtime and harvest, and cold and heat, and summer and winter, and day and night shall not cease [seedtime and harvest—giving first, then receiving]. (Gen. 8:22)

To order additional copies of

My
Personal Prayer
Journal

send $9.99 plus $3.95 shipping and handling to

Books, Etc.
PO Box 4888
Seattle, WA 98104

or have your credit card ready and call

(800) 917-BOOK